My Personal Diet & Meal Planner

Name : _____

Weight : _____

Goal Weight :

_____

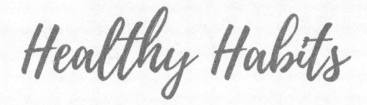

Healthy Habits

EAT HEALTHY MEALS

SHOP CONSCIOUSLY

GET ENOUGH SLEEP

EXERCISE FREQUENTLY

LAUGH OFTEN

SMILE

LOVE A LOT

BE KIND TO OTHERS

KEEP HYDRATED

WORK SMART

DO WHAT YOU LOVE

LEARN SOMETHING NEW

How to use this planner

YOU WILL FIND THAT YOUR WEIGHT LOSS AND
HEALTH GOALS WILL BE MORE ACHIEVABLE IF
YOU PLAN YOUR FOOD INTAKE EVERY DAY.
ADD SOME LIGHT EXERCISE, ENOUGH
HYDRATION AND SMALL HEALTHY SNACKS, AND
YOU WILL HAVE YOUR OWN WINNING RECIPE
FOR SUCCESS.

THIS PLANNER HELPS YOU TO DO THIS FOR
EACH DAY OVER 90 DAYS.
WITHIN THAT TIME YOU WILL DEVELOP LASTING
HEALTH HABITS THAT WILL BECOME YOUR
HEALTHY LIFESTYLE.

GOOD LUCK AND GIVE IT ALL YOU'VE GOT!

Meal Planner

DAY :

WATER INTAKE :

BREAKFAST

LUNCH

DINNER

HEALTHY SNACKS :

DAILY EXERCISE :

NOTES

NOTES

NOTES

NOTES

NOTES

Meal Planner

DAY :

NOTES

WATER INTAKE :

BREAKFAST

NOTES

LUNCH

NOTES

DINNER

NOTES

HEALTHY SNACKS :

NOTES

DAILY EXERCISE :

Meal Planner

DAY :

NOTES

WATER INTAKE :

BREAKFAST

NOTES

LUNCH

NOTES

DINNER

NOTES

HEALTHY SNACKS :

NOTES

DAILY EXERCISE :

Meal Planner

DAY :

WATER INTAKE :

BREAKFAST

LUNCH

DINNER

HEALTHY SNACKS :

DAILY EXERCISE :

NOTES

NOTES

NOTES

NOTES

NOTES

Meal Planner

DAY :

WATER INTAKE :

NOTES

BREAKFAST

NOTES

LUNCH

NOTES

DINNER

NOTES

HEALTHY SNACKS :

DAILY EXERCISE :

NOTES

Meal Planner

DAY :

BREAKFAST

LUNCH

DINNER

HEALTHY SNACKS :

DAILY EXERCISE :

NOTES

NOTES

NOTES

NOTES

NOTES

WATER INTAKE :

Meal Planner

DAY :

WATER INTAKE :

BREAKFAST

LUNCH

DINNER

HEALTHY SNACKS :

DAILY EXERCISE :

NOTES

NOTES

NOTES

NOTES

NOTES

Meal Planner

DAY :

NOTES

WATER INTAKE :

BREAKFAST

NOTES

LUNCH

NOTES

DINNER

NOTES

HEALTHY SNACKS :

NOTES

DAILY EXERCISE :

Meal Planner

DAY :

WATER INTAKE :

NOTES

BREAKFAST

NOTES

LUNCH

NOTES

DINNER

NOTES

HEALTHY SNACKS :

NOTES

DAILY EXERCISE :

Meal Planner

DAY :

NOTES

WATER INTAKE :

BREAKFAST

NOTES

LUNCH

NOTES

DINNER

NOTES

HEALTHY SNACKS :

NOTES

DAILY EXERCISE :

Meal Planner

DAY :

NOTES

WATER INTAKE :

BREAKFAST

NOTES

LUNCH

NOTES

DINNER

NOTES

HEALTHY SNACKS :

NOTES

DAILY EXERCISE :

Meal Planner

DAY :

WATER INTAKE :

BREAKFAST

LUNCH

DINNER

HEALTHY SNACKS :

DAILY EXERCISE :

NOTES

NOTES

NOTES

NOTES

NOTES

Meal Planner

DAY :

WATER INTAKE :

BREAKFAST

LUNCH

DINNER

HEALTHY SNACKS :

DAILY EXERCISE :

NOTES

NOTES

NOTES

NOTES

NOTES

Meal Planner

DAY :

WATER INTAKE :

NOTES

BREAKFAST

NOTES

LUNCH

NOTES

DINNER

NOTES

HEALTHY SNACKS :

NOTES

DAILY EXERCISE :

Meal Planner

DAY :

NOTES

WATER INTAKE :

BREAKFAST

NOTES

LUNCH

NOTES

DINNER

NOTES

HEALTHY SNACKS :

NOTES

DAILY EXERCISE :

Meal Planner

DAY :

WATER INTAKE :

BREAKFAST

LUNCH

DINNER

HEALTHY SNACKS :

DAILY EXERCISE :

NOTES

NOTES

NOTES

NOTES

NOTES

Meal Planner

DAY :

WATER INTAKE :

NOTES

BREAKFAST

NOTES

LUNCH

NOTES

DINNER

NOTES

HEALTHY SNACKS :

NOTES

DAILY EXERCISE :

Meal Planner

DAY :

NOTES

WATER INTAKE :

BREAKFAST

NOTES

LUNCH

NOTES

DINNER

NOTES

HEALTHY SNACKS :

NOTES

DAILY EXERCISE :

Meal Planner

DAY :

WATER INTAKE :

NOTES

BREAKFAST

NOTES

LUNCH

NOTES

DINNER

NOTES

HEALTHY SNACKS :

NOTES

DAILY EXERCISE :

Meal Planner

DAY :

NOTES

WATER INTAKE :

BREAKFAST

NOTES

LUNCH

NOTES

DINNER

NOTES

HEALTHY SNACKS :

NOTES

DAILY EXERCISE :

Meal Planner

DAY :

WATER INTAKE :

NOTES

BREAKFAST

NOTES

LUNCH

NOTES

DINNER

NOTES

HEALTHY SNACKS :

NOTES

DAILY EXERCISE :

Meal Planner

DAY :

WATER INTAKE :

NOTES

BREAKFAST

NOTES

LUNCH

NOTES

DINNER

NOTES

HEALTHY SNACKS :

NOTES

DAILY EXERCISE :

Meal Planner

DAY :

WATER INTAKE :

BREAKFAST

LUNCH

DINNER

HEALTHY SNACKS :

DAILY EXERCISE :

NOTES

NOTES

NOTES

NOTES

NOTES

Meal Planner

DAY :

WATER INTAKE :

BREAKFAST

LUNCH

DINNER

HEALTHY SNACKS :

DAILY EXERCISE :

NOTES

NOTES

NOTES

NOTES

NOTES

Meal Planner

DAY :

NOTES

WATER INTAKE :

BREAKFAST

NOTES

LUNCH

NOTES

DINNER

NOTES

HEALTHY SNACKS :

NOTES

DAILY EXERCISE :

Meal Planner

DAY :

WATER INTAKE :

BREAKFAST

LUNCH

DINNER

HEALTHY SNACKS :

DAILY EXERCISE :

NOTES

NOTES

NOTES

NOTES

NOTES

Meal Planner

DAY :

WATER INTAKE :

NOTES

BREAKFAST

NOTES

LUNCH

NOTES

DINNER

NOTES

HEALTHY SNACKS :

DAILY EXERCISE :

NOTES

Meal Planner

DAY :

NOTES

WATER INTAKE :

BREAKFAST

NOTES

LUNCH

NOTES

DINNER

NOTES

HEALTHY SNACKS :

NOTES

DAILY EXERCISE :

Meal Planner

DAY :

WATER INTAKE :

NOTES

BREAKFAST

NOTES

LUNCH

NOTES

DINNER

NOTES

HEALTHY SNACKS :

DAILY EXERCISE :

NOTES

Meal Planner

DAY :

WATER INTAKE :

NOTES

BREAKFAST

NOTES

LUNCH

NOTES

DINNER

NOTES

HEALTHY SNACKS :

DAILY EXERCISE :

NOTES

Meal Planner

DAY :

WATER INTAKE :

NOTES

BREAKFAST

NOTES

LUNCH

NOTES

DINNER

NOTES

HEALTHY SNACKS :

DAILY EXERCISE :

NOTES

Meal Planner

DAY :

NOTES

WATER INTAKE :

BREAKFAST

NOTES

LUNCH

NOTES

DINNER

NOTES

HEALTHY SNACKS :

NOTES

DAILY EXERCISE :

Meal Planner

DAY :

WATER INTAKE :

NOTES

BREAKFAST

NOTES

LUNCH

NOTES

DINNER

NOTES

HEALTHY SNACKS :

NOTES

DAILY EXERCISE :

Meal Planner

DAY :

WATER INTAKE :

NOTES

BREAKFAST

NOTES

LUNCH

NOTES

DINNER

NOTES

HEALTHY SNACKS :

NOTES

DAILY EXERCISE :

Meal Planner

DAY :

NOTES

WATER INTAKE :

BREAKFAST

NOTES

LUNCH

NOTES

DINNER

NOTES

HEALTHY SNACKS :

NOTES

DAILY EXERCISE :

Meal Planner

DAY :

WATER INTAKE :

BREAKFAST

LUNCH

DINNER

HEALTHY SNACKS :

DAILY EXERCISE :

NOTES

NOTES

NOTES

NOTES

NOTES

Meal Planner

DAY :

WATER INTAKE :

NOTES

BREAKFAST

NOTES

LUNCH

NOTES

DINNER

NOTES

HEALTHY SNACKS :

DAILY EXERCISE :

NOTES

Meal Planner

DAY :

WATER INTAKE :

BREAKFAST

LUNCH

DINNER

HEALTHY SNACKS :

DAILY EXERCISE :

NOTES

NOTES

NOTES

NOTES

NOTES

Meal Planner

DAY :

NOTES

WATER INTAKE :

BREAKFAST

NOTES

LUNCH

NOTES

DINNER

NOTES

HEALTHY SNACKS :

NOTES

DAILY EXERCISE :

Meal Planner

DAY :

WATER INTAKE :

BREAKFAST

LUNCH

DINNER

HEALTHY SNACKS :

DAILY EXERCISE :

NOTES

NOTES

NOTES

NOTES

NOTES

Meal Planner

DAY :

WATER INTAKE :

BREAKFAST

LUNCH

DINNER

HEALTHY SNACKS :

DAILY EXERCISE :

NOTES

NOTES

NOTES

NOTES

NOTES

Meal Planner

DAY :

WATER INTAKE :

NOTES

BREAKFAST

NOTES

LUNCH

NOTES

DINNER

NOTES

HEALTHY SNACKS :

NOTES

DAILY EXERCISE :

Meal Planner

DAY :

WATER INTAKE :

NOTES

BREAKFAST

NOTES

LUNCH

NOTES

DINNER

NOTES

HEALTHY SNACKS :

NOTES

DAILY EXERCISE :

Meal Planner

DAY :

WATER INTAKE :

BREAKFAST

LUNCH

DINNER

HEALTHY SNACKS :

DAILY EXERCISE :

NOTES

NOTES

NOTES

NOTES

NOTES

Meal Planner

DAY :

WATER INTAKE :

NOTES

BREAKFAST

NOTES

LUNCH

NOTES

DINNER

NOTES

HEALTHY SNACKS :

NOTES

DAILY EXERCISE :

Meal Planner

DAY :

WATER INTAKE :

NOTES

BREAKFAST

NOTES

LUNCH

NOTES

DINNER

NOTES

HEALTHY SNACKS :

NOTES

DAILY EXERCISE :

Meal Planner

DAY :

WATER INTAKE :

NOTES

BREAKFAST

NOTES

LUNCH

NOTES

DINNER

NOTES

HEALTHY SNACKS :

DAILY EXERCISE :

NOTES

Meal Planner

DAY :

WATER INTAKE :

BREAKFAST

LUNCH

DINNER

HEALTHY SNACKS :

DAILY EXERCISE :

NOTES

NOTES

NOTES

NOTES

NOTES

Meal Planner

DAY :

WATER INTAKE :

NOTES

BREAKFAST

NOTES

LUNCH

NOTES

DINNER

NOTES

HEALTHY SNACKS :

DAILY EXERCISE :

NOTES

Meal Planner

DAY :

WATER INTAKE :

BREAKFAST

LUNCH

DINNER

HEALTHY SNACKS :

DAILY EXERCISE :

NOTES

NOTES

NOTES

NOTES

NOTES

Meal Planner

DAY :

NOTES

WATER INTAKE :

BREAKFAST

NOTES

LUNCH

NOTES

DINNER

NOTES

HEALTHY SNACKS :

NOTES

DAILY EXERCISE :

Meal Planner

DAY :

NOTES

WATER INTAKE :

BREAKFAST

NOTES

LUNCH

NOTES

DINNER

NOTES

HEALTHY SNACKS :

NOTES

DAILY EXERCISE :

Meal Planner

DAY :

NOTES

WATER INTAKE :

BREAKFAST

NOTES

LUNCH

NOTES

DINNER

NOTES

HEALTHY SNACKS :

NOTES

DAILY EXERCISE :

Meal Planner

DAY :

WATER INTAKE :

BREAKFAST

LUNCH

DINNER

HEALTHY SNACKS :

DAILY EXERCISE :

NOTES

NOTES

NOTES

NOTES

NOTES

Meal Planner

DAY :

WATER INTAKE :

NOTES

BREAKFAST

NOTES

LUNCH

NOTES

DINNER

NOTES

HEALTHY SNACKS :

NOTES

DAILY EXERCISE :

Meal Planner

DAY :

NOTES

WATER INTAKE :

BREAKFAST

NOTES

LUNCH

NOTES

DINNER

NOTES

HEALTHY SNACKS :

NOTES

DAILY EXERCISE :

Meal Planner

DAY :

WATER INTAKE :

NOTES

BREAKFAST

NOTES

LUNCH

NOTES

DINNER

NOTES

HEALTHY SNACKS :

DAILY EXERCISE :

NOTES

Meal Planner

DAY :

WATER INTAKE :

BREAKFAST

LUNCH

DINNER

HEALTHY SNACKS :

DAILY EXERCISE :

NOTES

NOTES

NOTES

NOTES

NOTES

Meal Planner

DAY :

NOTES

WATER INTAKE :

BREAKFAST

NOTES

LUNCH

NOTES

DINNER

NOTES

HEALTHY SNACKS :

NOTES

DAILY EXERCISE :

Meal Planner

DAY :

WATER INTAKE :

NOTES

BREAKFAST

NOTES

LUNCH

NOTES

DINNER

NOTES

HEALTHY SNACKS :

NOTES

DAILY EXERCISE :

Meal Planner

DAY :

WATER INTAKE :

NOTES

BREAKFAST

NOTES

LUNCH

NOTES

DINNER

NOTES

HEALTHY SNACKS :

DAILY EXERCISE :

NOTES

Meal Planner

DAY :

WATER INTAKE :

BREAKFAST

LUNCH

DINNER

HEALTHY SNACKS :

DAILY EXERCISE :

NOTES

NOTES

NOTES

NOTES

NOTES

Meal Planner

DAY :

NOTES

WATER INTAKE :

BREAKFAST

NOTES

LUNCH

NOTES

DINNER

NOTES

HEALTHY SNACKS :

NOTES

DAILY EXERCISE :

Meal Planner

DAY :

WATER INTAKE :

NOTES

BREAKFAST

NOTES

LUNCH

NOTES

DINNER

NOTES

HEALTHY SNACKS :

NOTES

DAILY EXERCISE :

Meal Planner

DAY :

WATER INTAKE :

NOTES

BREAKFAST

NOTES

LUNCH

NOTES

DINNER

NOTES

HEALTHY SNACKS :

DAILY EXERCISE :

NOTES

Meal Planner

DAY :

NOTES

WATER INTAKE :

NOTES

BREAKFAST

NOTES

LUNCH

NOTES

DINNER

NOTES

HEALTHY SNACKS :

NOTES

DAILY EXERCISE :

Meal Planner

DAY :

NOTES

WATER INTAKE :

BREAKFAST

NOTES

LUNCH

NOTES

DINNER

NOTES

HEALTHY SNACKS :

NOTES

DAILY EXERCISE :

Meal Planner

DAY :

NOTES

WATER INTAKE :

NOTES

BREAKFAST

NOTES

LUNCH

NOTES

DINNER

NOTES

HEALTHY SNACKS :

NOTES

DAILY EXERCISE :

Meal Planner

DAY :

NOTES

WATER INTAKE :

BREAKFAST

NOTES

LUNCH

NOTES

DINNER

NOTES

HEALTHY SNACKS :

NOTES

DAILY EXERCISE :

Meal Planner

DAY :

NOTES

WATER INTAKE :

NOTES

BREAKFAST

NOTES

LUNCH

NOTES

DINNER

NOTES

HEALTHY SNACKS :

NOTES

DAILY EXERCISE :

Meal Planner

DAY :

WATER INTAKE :

NOTES

BREAKFAST

NOTES

LUNCH

NOTES

DINNER

NOTES

HEALTHY SNACKS :

DAILY EXERCISE :

NOTES

Meal Planner

DAY :

WATER INTAKE :

BREAKFAST

LUNCH

DINNER

HEALTHY SNACKS :

DAILY EXERCISE :

NOTES

NOTES

NOTES

NOTES

NOTES

Meal Planner

DAY :

WATER INTAKE :

NOTES

BREAKFAST

NOTES

LUNCH

NOTES

DINNER

NOTES

HEALTHY SNACKS :

DAILY EXERCISE :

NOTES

Meal Planner

DAY :

WATER INTAKE :

BREAKFAST

LUNCH

DINNER

HEALTHY SNACKS :

DAILY EXERCISE :

NOTES

NOTES

NOTES

NOTES

NOTES

Meal Planner

DAY :

WATER INTAKE :

BREAKFAST

LUNCH

DINNER

HEALTHY SNACKS :

DAILY EXERCISE :

NOTES

NOTES

NOTES

NOTES

NOTES

Meal Planner

DAY :

WATER INTAKE :

BREAKFAST

LUNCH

DINNER

HEALTHY SNACKS :

DAILY EXERCISE :

NOTES

NOTES

NOTES

NOTES

NOTES

NOTES

Meal Planner

DAY :

NOTES

WATER INTAKE :

BREAKFAST

NOTES

LUNCH

NOTES

DINNER

NOTES

HEALTHY SNACKS :

NOTES

DAILY EXERCISE :

Meal Planner

DAY :

NOTES

WATER INTAKE :

NOTES

BREAKFAST

NOTES

LUNCH

NOTES

DINNER

NOTES

HEALTHY SNACKS :

NOTES

DAILY EXERCISE :

Meal Planner

DAY :

WATER INTAKE :

NOTES

BREAKFAST

NOTES

LUNCH

NOTES

DINNER

NOTES

HEALTHY SNACKS :

DAILY EXERCISE :

NOTES

Meal Planner

DAY :

WATER INTAKE :

BREAKFAST

LUNCH

DINNER

HEALTHY SNACKS :

DAILY EXERCISE :

NOTES

NOTES

NOTES

NOTES

NOTES

Meal Planner

DAY :

WATER INTAKE :

NOTES

BREAKFAST

NOTES

LUNCH

NOTES

DINNER

NOTES

HEALTHY SNACKS :

NOTES

DAILY EXERCISE :

Meal Planner

DAY :

WATER INTAKE :

BREAKFAST

LUNCH

DINNER

HEALTHY SNACKS :

DAILY EXERCISE :

NOTES

NOTES

NOTES

NOTES

NOTES

Meal Planner

DAY :

NOTES

WATER INTAKE :

BREAKFAST

NOTES

LUNCH

NOTES

DINNER

NOTES

HEALTHY SNACKS :

NOTES

DAILY EXERCISE :

Meal Planner

DAY :

WATER INTAKE :

BREAKFAST

LUNCH

DINNER

HEALTHY SNACKS :

DAILY EXERCISE :

NOTES

NOTES

NOTES

NOTES

NOTES

Meal Planner

DAY :

WATER INTAKE :

NOTES

BREAKFAST

NOTES

LUNCH

NOTES

DINNER

NOTES

HEALTHY SNACKS :

NOTES

DAILY EXERCISE :

Meal Planner

DAY :

WATER INTAKE :

BREAKFAST

LUNCH

DINNER

HEALTHY SNACKS :

DAILY EXERCISE :

NOTES

NOTES

NOTES

NOTES

NOTES

Meal Planner

DAY :

WATER INTAKE :

NOTES

BREAKFAST

NOTES

LUNCH

NOTES

DINNER

NOTES

HEALTHY SNACKS :

NOTES

DAILY EXERCISE :

Meal Planner

DAY :

NOTES

WATER INTAKE :

NOTES

BREAKFAST

NOTES

LUNCH

NOTES

DINNER

NOTES

HEALTHY SNACKS :

NOTES

DAILY EXERCISE :

Meal Planner

DAY :

WATER INTAKE :

NOTES

BREAKFAST

NOTES

LUNCH

NOTES

DINNER

NOTES

HEALTHY SNACKS :

NOTES

DAILY EXERCISE :

Meal Planner

DAY :

WATER INTAKE :

BREAKFAST

LUNCH

DINNER

HEALTHY SNACKS :

DAILY EXERCISE :

NOTES

NOTES

NOTES

NOTES

NOTES

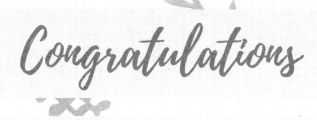

Congratulations

CONGRATULATIONS ON YOUR ACHIEVEMENTS.

WRITE YOUR THOUGHTS AND IDEAS THAT YOU HAVE LEARNED ALONG THE WAY - THINGS THAT WILL HELP YOU TO KEEP YOUR HEALTHY LIFESTYLE.

Notes & Ideas

Notes & Ideas

Notes & Ideas

Notes & Ideas

Notes & Ideas

Notes & Ideas

Made in the USA
Columbia, SC
18 January 2020